10 DAY
HEALTHY LIFESTYLE
CHALLENGE

CRISTINA DOMINGOS

10 DAY HEALTHY LIFESTYLE CHALLENGE

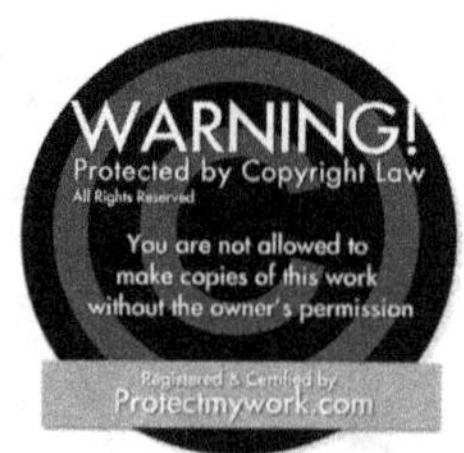

🙰🙰

"Please test us for ten days on a diet of vegetables and water," Daniel said. At the end of the ten days, see how we look compared to the other young men who are eating the king's food. Then make your decision in light of what you see.The attendant agreed to Daniel's suggestion and tested them for ten days."

−Daniel 1:12−14 NLT

Contents

1
Introduction

5
Prayer

6
My Healthy Life Journey

9
Reduce Toxic Chemicals In Your Body and Home

11
Cleansing Your Organs To Stay Healthy.

13
Reduce Exposure To Air Pollution

15
A Healthy Sleep Pattern

17
Prayer To Be Born Again and To Receive Jesus Christ as Your Lord and Savior

19
Lord, Teach Me To live According To Your Precepts

21
Biblical Declaration For A Peaceful Sleep

23
10 Day Healthy Lifestyle Challenge Protocol

25
Bible Verses About Healthy Lifestyle To Meditate

38
Reflection Of The Challenge

40
Acknowledgements

41
About The Author

Introduction

Welcome to the 10-day healthy lifestyle challenge! This book will encourage you to adopt a healthier way of living. We all only have one body and must take good care of it. It's time for us to evaluate what we consume. Poor dietary choices can lead to preventable diseases. If we consistently consume unhealthy fast food instead of healthy meals, our bodies and overall health will pay for it later. As born-again Christians, we are the temple of the Holy Spirit (1 Corinthians 6:19). We must, therefore, care for our bodies and be mindful of what we eat. We must continually assess our diets. Are they beneficial, or are they harmful? Do they have the potential to cause illnesses? Some foods are like medicine, and others are just pure poison. We do not want to put poison in the temple of the Holy Spirit. Let's keep in mind that not just the food we eat can be toxic; the products we use on our skin can also negatively affect our health. Many people are not aware of this fact. If we focus solely on eating healthy but continue to use skin products that contain toxic ingredients, we are not fully living a healthy lifestyle.

If we observe carefully, many products on our shelves are harmful or contain harmful elements. As a result, some things will be beyond our control. However, there are numerous things that we can change to reduce the toxicity in our lives. The rest we have to leave it in God's hands. Isaiah 54:17 is a beautiful scripture that reads: "No weapon formed against me shall prosper."

You may be wondering why I say a lot of products are toxic. Well, we live in a fallen world, and satan is the "god" of this world. His mission is to kill, steal and destroy, and how better to achieve his aim than to make sure we get sick through using everyday products? I acknowledge that people create these things, but we do not wrestle against flesh and blood (Ephesians 6:12). The devil uses people to accomplish his mission.

Make sure you always read the labels before you buy a product. Do this, not just for yourself but also for your babies. Not all baby products are natural; some contain parfum and other chemicals. Beware, not all products marked "natural" are. They may have "natural" in the front, but if you read the back of the products, they have "parfum" or "fragrance" as one of the ingredients. In addition, avoid any product with "Synthetic Fragrances" written on it. That one ingredient contains many hidden toxic chemicals. The bottom line is always avoid parfum, even if the product says biologic, organic, or natural. The fewer ingredients in a product, the better. Sometimes it's hard to find natural products in normal grocery stores. You can order them online or buy them in organic stores. Most importantly, pray over everything you buy from the stores, market, etc. Ask God to sanctify everything you buy with the Blood of Jesus, no matter what it is.

There are so many benefits of eating healthy food:

- You will have more energy for more activities throughout the day.

- Your skin will glow and look healthier.

- You will sleep better.

- Eating healthy food can contribute to a longer life for you.

- You will not go to the doctor often, saving you money in doctor's fees.

- You will think more clearly.

- Your moods may improve by eating less processed foods.

- You can lose weight.

In this 10-Day Healthy Lifestyle Challenge, you will eat healthier for ten consecutive days and exercise at least 3-4 times a week. For this challenge, you will not be eating any animal products. You can read on the 10-Day Healthy Food Challenge Protocol what foods you should avoid. During this period, you will examine your home products to see if they are harmful. Read the labels and do your research.

You can start any day you want or do this challenge every month. It may seem challenging, but Christ will give you the strength to finish. Plan the meals you want to eat to simplify your grocery shopping. Plan your meals using the planner included in this book.

Eating healthy does not have to be expensive. A word of advice, include the whole family. It is good to start the children early so that they get used to eating healthy food. Children like eating sweet things like candy, chocolate, etc. Artificial food dyes can also be harmful to children. There may be a link between food dyes and hyperactivity in children. If you have hyperactive children, consider cutting off all snacks with artificial food dyes for more than a week and see if there are changes in their behavior. These food coloring agents are found in candies, brightly colored cereals, and sugary cake decorations, among other things. Explain to your children why you are doing it, and ensure you reward them if they participate in the challenge. We are living in the last days, and the enemy is after our children. He wants to destroy them so that when they grow up, they will not be able to walk in the destiny God has for them.

You can also do the challenge with a friend or a colleague.

To succeed in this challenge, you will have to come out of your comfort zone. May the Lord give you the strength you need to complete this challenge. Your body will definitely thank you for it.

Prayer

Dear Heavenly Father,

I come before You through Your precious Son, Jesus Christ. I need Your help to change my lifestyle. I recognize that my body is the temple of the Holy Spirit, and I am not my own. I was bought with a high price. I want to honor You with my body by taking care of it. Lord, I ask You to forgive me for not caring for my body by eating harmful food. I am grateful for the body You have given me and for providing for me daily. Everything You have created is good. Thank You for vegetables and fruits because they are like medicine to my body. With Your help, I will eat them so that my body is nourished with the vitamins, minerals, and fiber it needs. Lord, I want to glorify You in everything I do, including nutrition and exercise. I know Your will for me is to stay healthy and have a sound mind so that I accomplish Your will for my life. Lord, give me the wisdom and discernment to know which foods are good for my family and I and which are bad. Lord, reveal to me any toxic product I have in my home that I need to dispose of. I do not want to do this challenge in my own strength. I need You. Today, I declare that I can do all things through Christ Who gives me strength.

I give You all the honor and glory.

In Jesus' name I pray,

Amen

My Healthy Life Journey

My healthy lifestyle journey began in 2016 before I started nursing school. I decided to eat healthy and less processed food. I also started going to the gym. I never liked working out, so this was a challenge for me. In 2019, I started with my natural journey, switching certain products to natural ones.

I used to have heart palpitations but did not know what the cause was. I went to a doctor who referred me to a hospital where I received a Holter heart monitor that recorded my heart activity for 24 hours. After analyzing the results, they could not detect anything unusual. The doctors advised me not to worry about it. One day I was on a live stream; a sister in Christ was praying for people, and she also prayed for me. Nothing happened, but she gave me a word. She said that the Lord would teach me things concerning my healing. I continued praying about my health and discovered I was allergic to MSG (E621). MSG is a flavor enhancer that they add to many food products, like canned food, pizza, some packaged food, and many more. It was the reason I had these heart palpitations. I thank God for revealing that to me. I noticed that when I stopped eating certain foods, the heart palpitations also stopped. All glory to the Most High. This incident prompted me to start reading food labels on food products that I was purchasing. I knew that if a food product contained E621, I could not buy it.

In 2021, I did more research on natural products. In 2019 I had switched certain products like deodorant and toothpaste to natural ones, but that was about it. I continued my research and started using more natural cleaning and washing products. Since my journey began in 2016, I have learned so much.

Unknown to me, I was vitamin D deficient. I found out when the doctor did some blood tests. My vitamin D level in my blood was 17 ng/ml which is extremely low. The doctor said that it needed to be around 50 ng/ml. The problem is that many people are deficient and are not aware. This condition is especially prevalent for people of color because it is not as easy for dark-skinned people to make vitamin D from the sunlight, those above 65 years, and people who do not regularly go outside. Vitamin D is essential for our immune system. Being deficient in it can cause other diseases. That is why it is an essential vitamin.

I also used to be chronically tired without knowing why. The cause, I later found out, was a vitamin D deficiency. The doctor prescribed vitamin D for me to get from the pharmacy. Because I had cultivated a habit of always reading the labels, I was curious to find out what was in the vitamin D. The one prescribed contained two E numbers, E129 and E110. Of course, I did my research! E129 is a red dye, and I discovered that it could cause allergies or irritations like headaches, dizziness, hyperactivity in children, etc. E110 could also cause allergic reactions such as hormonal changes, allergies, kidney problems, migraines, etc. I called the pharmacy and asked them if they had one without the E numbers. I decided to search for one without preservatives and synthetic colors. I now use natural vegan vitamin oils. We have one body, and it is our responsibility to research the products we put in our bodies.

Be sure to measure your vitamin D. Often, people have many health issues because of the lack of vitamins and minerals. We don't always need to take pills for everything. Find out the root cause before taking any. It could be a minor issue like what I had, food allergies, and vitamin deficiency. Just imagine if the doctor had prescribed heart medication. It would not have solved the problem but made it worse because the root cause needed to be addressed. Fortunately, we serve a living God who reveals all hidden things. Amen. There are many diseases we can avoid if we eat more healthy food.

Reduce Toxic Chemicals In Your Body and Home

Here are 10 products that I have swapped for natural alternatives.

1. Toothpaste: I have switched to natural options that have fewer ingredients.

2. Deodorant: Many deodorants contain aluminum. It's best to use those without it. Many stores now sell alum-free deodorant.

3. Shampoo, conditioner, and hair creams: Use sulfate-free shampoos and natural hair products.

4. Body lotion: I disposed of all my body lotions because they had many harmful ingredients. I now only use olive oil. It is very healthy for the skin and contains antioxidants. Olive oil is also a biblical oil; used by people in bible times. Psalm 104:15 reads, "Olive oil for our skin, and grain for our health."

5. Hand soaps: Most hand soaps contain sulfate and synthetic fragrances which have many hidden chemicals. We should avoid using them because we wash our hands several times daily. Every time we do, those ingredients enter our bodies.

6. Menstrual pads: Many menstrual pads have harmful chemicals and fragrances. These ingredients can make a period worse. Toxic pads can contribute to heavy and painful menstrual cramps. I highly recommend that girls and women consider

using organic cotton pads instead. You can find organic pads in stores that sell organic products. If buying organic pads is difficult, reusable pads are a good option. They are washable and reusable.

7. Vitamin supplements: We all need vitamins to keep our bodies healthy. There are so many options on the market. Some vitamins contact harmful chemicals. Do not think just because they are vitamins, they are healthy. Just like other products, there are good and bad ones. Always read the labels.

8. Dishwashers: Buy non-toxic dishwashers.

9. Laundry detergents: Many laundry detergents that we use contain harmful chemicals. They remain in our clothes and also come into contact with our skin. That is why it is important to buy natural laundry detergents.

10. Cleaning products: I now use organic alternatives that do not contain toxic chemicals.

Cleansing Your Organs To Stay Healthy.

We make sure we take showers and baths every day to keep ourselves clean and smelling good. However, we often neglect to cleanse the inside of our bodies. Consuming unhealthy food can be very harmful to our bodies. Sickness doesn't happen overnight; it accumulates over time. It may even take years before someone becomes ill.

We may have to deal with the consequences of our actions today, much later. Our bodies will thank us later if we nourish them with healthy and nutritious food. It is amazing how God made our bodies. They can heal themselves if we let them. For instance, when we experience a fall or a cut, the wound eventually closes and heals on its own.

Our lymphatic system plays a vital role in our health. We could have gotten sick many times, but the lymphatic system ensures that toxins are eliminated from our bodies. However, certain factors can hinder its proper functioning, causing it to become sluggish or clogged.

Our lymphatic system plays a vital role in our health. We could have gotten sick many times, but the lymphatic system ensures that toxins are eliminated from our bodies. However, certain factors can hinder its proper functioning, causing it to become sluggish or clogged.

Things you should do to avoid lymphatic system blockage:

- Eat less processed and sugary food.

- Drink enough water throughout the day.

- Exercise at least 3-4 times a week.

- Stop habitually wearing tight clothes like skinny jeans, tight underwear, etc. Tight clothes can cause poor blood circulation.

- Wear bras without an underwire, and avoid sleeping with a bra.

- Try using castor oil for cleansing purposes, using organic castor oil that comes in a glass container. This pack can help detoxify your body and boost your immune system. I suggest that you conduct some research on this topic as castor oil offers many health benefits.

Reduce Exposure
To Air Pollution

Considering the multitudes of toxins we inhale daily from our environment, we need to remove toxic substances from our bodies. Both outdoor and indoor settings expose us to harmful substances like air pollution from transportation, house cleaning products, perfume, cigarette, paint, scented candles, air freshener, deodorant, hair spray, etc. Prolonged exposure to polluted air can negatively affect the health of our bodies. It can also lead to the accumulation of heavy metals in our bodies. Fortunately, there are actions we can take to minimize our exposure and safeguard our well-being.

Here are some actions you can implement to get you started:

1   Drink lemon water. Lemons contain a lot of vitamin C.

2   Buy air-purifying plants for your home.

3   Use aroma diffusers instead of candles. Use 100% natural essential oils containing only one or two ingredients. And if you want to use candles, choose candles without paraffin. For example, you can choose soy and beeswax candles. These candles are a bit more expensive in price, though.

4   Drink green juices to remove toxins, like heavy metal from your body. Make your own, and not store-bought. Green juices that are good for removing heavy metals from your body are:

5 Green juices that are good for removing heavy metals from your body are:

- Parsley with lemon
- Coriander juice
- Cucumber juice
- Spinach along with carrot juice

6 Eat fruits that contain antioxidants. Fruits like berries, especially; blueberries, are rich in antioxidants. You can eat fruits as they are or make juice or smoothies with them.

7 Buy a water filter. It will remove microplastics, chlorine, heavy metals, medicine, hormones, bacteria, and other toxic substances from your water. The added benefit is that you won't need to buy bottled water.

8 Change your cleaning products.

9 Clean your home regularly. Don't let dust accumulate in your home, especially your bedroom.

10 Open your windows every morning.

11 Don't stand near someone who is smoking.

A Healthy Sleep Pattern

good and healthy sleep pattern is also part of a healthy lifestyle. The average adult sleep requirement is 6-8 hours per night. Sleep is very important to us. Unfortunately, many people struggle with sleep problems. Sleepless nights can be caused by many things such as : Stress, phone/social media, worrying about children, problems, worrying about the future, heavy meals before bedtime, going to bed late, lack of good vitamins in diet, sleeping where there is a lot of noise, illnesses, drinking caffeinated beverages such as cola, tea, coffee, energy drinks.

During our sleep our immune systems are strengthened, our bodies are refreshed, it's good for our brain, heart, lung, we get the rest we need and God speaks to us in our dreams.

Sleep is a blessing given to us by our Dear Heavenly Father God, all His children should have a good night's sleep. No matter what happens in our lives, but not all Christians experience this sleep.

Things you can do to get a good night sleep:

1. Give your life to the Lord Jesus, let Him lead in your life. If you have not yet given your life to the Lord Jesus, I invite you to pray the salvation prayer.

2. Prayer, before going to bed. Praying before bed is very important, prayer becomes even more powerful when you take the Word of God and proclaim and pray His Word. Bible texts you could proclaim every dg before bed are Psalm 4:8,Psalm 23, Psalm 91, Psalm 121, speak them out loud. Thank God for the day you have had.

3   Never go to bed without repenting of your sins, you should do this every day/night. And forgive everyone who has hurt you.

4   Read the Bible before you go to sleep. And possibly have Bible audio on for the whole night. This way your mind will hear the word of God. You can download a bible app on your mobile phone for free.

5   1 hour before bedtime don't look at social media when you are in bed, don't watch TV or go on the computer. The light that is in those screens will prevent you to go to sleep early.

6   Make sure that you get enough vitamin B6, B3 And B12 through a healthy diet

7   Do not drink coffee or green- black tea before bedtime. Avoid drinking alcohol.

8   Making sure the bedroom is cleaned regularly.

9   Avoid using sleeping medicine, they can cause other side effects,

10   Drink sleep-inducing tea, such as chamomile, lavender and mint tea. Drink this about 1 hour to half an hour before going to bed. Caution! If you are taking medication, then you should check carefully if you can drink this tea.

11   Turn on a diffuser in your bedroom 1 hour or half an hour before you go to sleep. Lavender is a good essential oil that you can use for good sleep rest. Make sure the lavender is 100% natural with no other added ingredients.

12   Do not watch horror movie or other scary movies. By watching these movies you open doors for bad spirits. These bad spirits can disturb your sleep. I won't go into much detail here, but as you grow in your faith, God will reveal more things to you.

13   Go to bed at a set time.

Prayer To Be Born Again and To Receive Jesus Christ as Your Lord and Savior

Jesus answered and said to him, "Most assuredly, I say to you, **unless** one is **born again**, he cannot see the kingdom of God."

Nicodemus said to Him, "How can a man be born when he is old? Can he enter a second time into his mother's womb and be born?"

Jesus answered, "Most assuredly, I say to you, unless one is **born of water and the Spirit**, he cannot enter the kingdom of God. That which is born of the flesh is flesh, and that which is born of the Spirit is spirit. Do not marvel that I said to you, **'You must be born again.'**

– John 3:3-7

Dear Heavenly Father,

I admit that I am a sinner. I have done many things that do not please You. I have lived my life for myself only. I am sorry, and I repent, Lord I ask You to forgive me. I believe, confess and acknowledge that Jesus Christ is the Son of God, who died on the cross and rose on the third day, to save me. For Your Word in *Romans* 10:9 declares that if I confess with my mouth, that "Jesus is Lord," and believe in my heart that God raised him from the dead, I will be saved. Lord, I am very grateful. I receive Jesus as my Lord and Savior.

Jesus said in *John* 3:3 that unless a person is born again (reborn from above, spiritually, transformed, renewed and sanctified) that he cannot ever see and experience the Kingdom of God. Lord, I want to be born again I want to experience Your Kingdom. I want to leave my past behind , be born of water and the Spirit and follow the Lord Jesus Chris. Lord, sprinkle clean water on me and I will be clean. Cleanse me from all my uncleanness and from my idols. I want to change my old way of thinking, returning from my sinful ways and to change my life because I love You and I do not want to perish.

Remove the stony heart from my body and replace it with a heart that's God-willed and not self willed. Lord, put Your Spirit in me and make it possible for me to do what You tell me and to live by Your commands. I will be Yours and You will be my God. I want to be lead by Your Spirit, so that I may call myself a child of God. Because Your Word in *Romans* 8:14 declares that all who are allowing themselves to be led by the Spirit of God are sons of God. Lord, help me to take my everyday, my ordinary life, my sleeping, my eating, going to work and walking around and place it before You as an offering. Help me to fix my attention to You. So that I may be changed form the inside out. Lord, bring the best out of me, develop a well-formed maturity in me. I come to You now and ask You to take control of my life; Lord I give it to You. Lord, help me from this day forward, live every day for You and in a way that pleases You.

I give You all the glory and honor.

In Jesus' name I pray,

Amen

Lord, Teach Me To live According To Your Precepts

Dear Heavenly Father,

I will praise You with an upright heart, as I learn Your righteous laws. I can only stay on the patch of purity, by living according to Your word. I will seek You with all my heart everyday of my life. Praise be to You, Lord, teach me Your decrees. Lord open my eyes so that I may see the wonderful things in Your law. Lord, Keep me from deceitful ways, be gracious to me and teach me Your law. Teach me, Lord, the way of Your decrees, that I may follow it to the end. Give me understanding, so that I may keep Your law and obey it with all my heart. Direct me in the path of Your commands, for there I find delight. Before I was afflicted I went astray, but now I obey Your word. You are good, and what You do is good, teach me Your decrees. Your hands made me and formed me, give me understanding to learn Your commands. If Your law had not been my delight, I would have perished in my affliction. I have kept my feet from every evil path, so that I might obey Your Word. I have not departed from Your laws, for You Yourself have taught me. Your Word is a lamp to my feet, a light on my path. I have taken an oath and confirmed it, that I will follow your righteous laws.You are my refuge and my shield, I have put my hope in Your word. Sustain me, my God, according to Your promise, and I will live, do not let my hopes be dashed.Direct my footsteps according to Your words, let no sin rule over me. You are righteous, Lord, and Your laws are right. Your righteousness is everlasting and Your law is true. I call with all my heart; answer me, Lord, and I will obey Your decrees. I call out to you; save me and I will keep Your statutes. Hear my voice in accordance with Your love; preserve my life, Lord, according to Your laws. Great peace have those who love Your law, and nothing can make them stumble. I wait for Your salvation, Lord, and I follow Your commands. I obey Your statutes, for I love them greatly.

In Jesus' Name I pray,

Amen

Biblical Declaration For A Peaceful Sleep

In peace, I will both lie down and sleep; for you alone, O Lord, make me dwell in safety, according to Psalms 4:8.

⬰⬱

I declare that when I lie down, my sleep will be sweet, according to Proverbs 3:24.

⬰⬱

I lay down and slept, I woke again, for the Lord sustained me, according to Psalms 3:5.

⬰⬱

I will lay my labor and heavy laden, and the Lord will give me rest, according to Matthew 11:28.

⬰⬱

The Lord will cause a deep sleep to fall upon me, according to Genesis 2:21.

⬰⬱

I declare that my sleep will be pleasant to me, according to Jeremiah 31:26.

⬰⬱

I declare that I will not be anxious about tomorrow, for tomorrow will be anxious for itself, according to Matthew 6:34.

⬰⬱

I will cast all my anxieties on the Lord, because He cares for me, according to 1 Peter 5:7.

ℰℭ

I will lay down and none will make me afraid, according to Job 11:19.

ℰℭ

The Lord's presence will go with me and He will give me rest, according to Exodus 33:14.

ℰℭ

For the Lord gives me sleep, according to Psalms 127:2.

ℰℭ

On His law I meditate day and night, according to Psalms 1:2.

ℰℭ

The Lord has left peace with me, His peace He gave me. He does not give to me as the world gives, according to John 14:27.

ℰℭ

For the Lord has not given me a spirit of fear, but a spirit of love, and of power, and a sound mind. To live each day and glorify His name, according to 2 Timothy 1:7.

ℰℭ

The peace of God, which transcends all understanding, will guard my heart and my mind in Christ Jesus, according Phillipians 4:7.

10 Day Healthy Lifestyle Challenge Protocol

Foods to avoid during this ten day challenge:	Drinks to avoid during this ten day challenge:	What foods to eat during this ten day food challenge:	What can you drink during this ten day food challenge:
All animal products, including meat, fish, cheese, milk, eggs, margarine	Coffee	Fresh or frozen vegetables	Water. If you like flavored water you can add slices of lemon, lime, cucumber, fresh mint leaves, orange, strawberries, etc.
Fast Food	Soda	Fruits	Flavoured water. You can add slices of lemon, lime, cucumber, fresh mint leaves, orange, strawberries, etc.
Candy, Cookies, cake, ice cream	Fruit Juices bought in stores(some of these juices contains a lot of sugar)	Irish potatoes, sweet potatoes, purple potatoes	Tea without sugar
Chips	Energy drinks	Brown rice , red rice, wild rice, and black rice.	Homemade smoothies: Fruit smoothies, Green Smoothies.

Foods to avoid during this ten day challenge:	Drinks to avoid during this ten day challenge:	What foods to eat during this ten day food challenge:	What can you drink during this ten day food challenge:
Pasta	Sweetened tea	Unsalted Nuts	Homemade juices: Fruit juices, vegetable juices like celery juice (drink on empty stomach).
Sugar	Store bought Smoothies	Oatmeal	
Pizza	Sports drinks	Beans and legume	
sugary breakfast cereals,	Store bought vitamine water		
Canned food			
White bread			
White rice

Instant noodles. | | | |
| Chinese food | | | |

Be creative and search the internet for meals without animal products. You will find many recipes, including various smoothies and juice recipes.

Bible Verses About Healthy Lifestyle To Meditate

"Or do you not know that your body is a temple of the Holy Spirit within you, whom you have from God? You are not your own, for you were bought with a price. So glorify God in your body."

-1 Corinthians 6:19-20

☯

"So, *whether you eat or drink*, or whatever you do, do all to the glory of God."

-1 Corinthians 10:31

☯

If anyone *destroys God's temple*, God will destroy him. For God's temple is holy, and you are that temple.

-1 Corinthians 3:17

☯

"Beloved, I pray that all may go well with you and that you may be in good health, as it goes well with your soul.

-3 John 1:2

☯

"I appeal to you therefore, brothers, by the mercies of God, to present your bodies as a living sacrifice, holy and acceptable to God, which is your spiritual worship. Do not be conformed to this world, but be transformed by the renewal of your mind, that by testing you may discern what is the will of God, what is good and acceptable and perfect."

— Romans 12:1-2

৪৩

"And God said, "Behold, I have given you every plant yielding seed that is on the face of all the earth, and every tree with seed in its fruit. You shall have them for food."

— Genesis 1:29

৪৩

A joyful heart is good medicine, but a crushed spirit dries up the bones.

—Proverbs 17:22

৪৩

"No temptation has overtaken you that is not common to man. God is faithful, and he will not let you be tempted beyond your ability, but with the temptation he will also provide the way of escape, that you may be able to endure it."

1 Corinthians 10:13

৪৩

"Every moving thing that lives shall be food for you. And as I gave you the green plants, I give you everything."

—Genesis 9:3

୫୦୯ଷ

"And you will know the truth, and the truth will set you free."

— John 8:32

୫୦୯ଷ

Nor thieves, nor the greedy, *nor drunkards*, nor revilers, nor swindlers will inherit the kingdom of God.

—1 Corinthians 6:10

୫୦୯ଷ

"Do not be anxious about anything, but in everything by prayer and supplication with thanksgiving let your requests be made known to God. And the peace of God, which surpasses all understanding, will guard your hearts and your minds in Christ Jesus."

—Philippians 4:6-7

| DAILY PLANNER OF ________________ | DATE: |

| I am grateful for |

MEALS

| BREAKFAST | LUNCH | DINNER |

THINGS TO DO

| MORNING | AFTERNOON | EVENING |

10 DAY HEALTHY LIFESTYLE CHALLENGE PLANNER

| DAILY PLANNER OF ___________________ | DATE: |

I am grateful for

MEALS

| BREAKFAST | LUNCH | DINNER |

THINGS TO DO

| MORNING | AFTERNOON | EVENING |

10 DAY HEALTHY LIFESTYLE CHALLENGE
PLANNER

DAILY PLANNER OF _____________________ | DATE:

I am grateful for

MEALS

| BREAKFAST | LUNCH | DINNER |

THINGS TO DO

| MORNING | AFTERNOON | EVENING |

10 DAY HEALTHY LIFESTYLE CHALLENGE PLANNER

<table>
<tr><td>DAILY PLANNER OF _______________________</td><td>DATE:</td></tr>
</table>

I am grateful for

MEALS

BREAKFAST	LUNCH	DINNER

THINGS TO DO

MORNING	AFTERNOON	EVENING

10 DAY HEALTHY LIFESTYLE CHALLENGE
PLANNER

<table>
<tr><td>DAILY PLANNER OF ________________________</td><td>DATE:</td></tr>
</table>

I am grateful for

MEALS

BREAKFAST	LUNCH	DINNER

THINGS TO DO

MORNING	AFTERNOON	EVENING

10 DAY HEALTHY LIFESTYLE CHALLENGE PLANNER

| DAILY PLANNER OF ________________________ | DATE: |

I am grateful for

MEALS

| BREAKFAST | LUNCH | DINNER |

THINGS TO DO

| MORNING | AFTERNOON | EVENING |

10 DAY HEALTHY LIFESTYLE CHALLENGE
PLANNER

DAILY PLANNER OF _________________	DATE:

I am grateful for

MEALS

BREAKFAST	LUNCH	DINNER

THINGS TO DO

MORNING	AFTERNOON	EVENING

10 DAY HEALTHY LIFESTYLE CHALLENGE PLANNER

| DAILY PLANNER OF _____________________ | DATE: |

I am grateful for

MEALS

| BREAKFAST | LUNCH | DINNER |

THINGS TO DO

| MORNING | AFTERNOON | EVENING |

10 DAY HEALTHY LIFESTYLE CHALLENGE PLANNER

| DAILY PLANNER OF _______________________ | DATE: |

I am grateful for

MEALS

| BREAKFAST | LUNCH | DINNER |

THINGS TO DO

| MORNING | AFTERNOON | EVENING |

10 DAY HEALTHY LIFESTYLE CHALLENGE PLANNER

| DAILY PLANNER OF ___________________ | DATE: |

I am grateful for

MEALS

| BREAKFAST | LUNCH | DINNER |

THINGS TO DO

| MORNING | AFTERNOON | EVENING |

10 DAY HEALTHY LIFESTYLE CHALLENGE
PLANNER

Reflection Of The Challenge

Congratulations, you have finished the
10-day healthy lifestyle challenge!

◈ What changes have you noticed during the ten-day healthy lifestyle challenge?

❖ What food and drinks will you cut off for good, and what will you add to?

____

____

____

____

____

____

❖ Which products are you going to switch to a natural one?

____

____

____

____

____

____

____

Acknowledgements

I give all the honor and glory to God the Father, Jesus Christ, the Son of God, and the Holy Spirit, my Helper. I would not be able to write this book, without God. I let God use my hand as His pen to write the message to the people that He wants to reach. I thank God for giving me the strength and the courage to write this book, because I know that's what He has called me to do. It's not by my might, not by my power, but by His Spirit.

I thank God for sending His only begotten son Jesus Christ for all of us so that we can have a relationship with Him. Thank You Jesus. I pray that this book will help people to live a healthy lifestyle, a lifestyle that will glorify the Lord.

I thank God for using me as His vessel for His Kingdom, and I pray that He may continue to use me. For the Spirit of the Lord God is upon me, because He has anointed and commissioned me to bring good news to the humble and afflicted.

He has sent me to bind up wounds of the brokenhearted, to proclaim release from confinement and condemnation to the physical and spiritual captives. There is no one like Jesus Christ and I thank my Lord for everything He has done, for what He is doing and for what He will do. God is good. In Jesus name Amen

About The Author

Cristina Domingos is a born-again believer and the author of "GOD'S PERFECT WILL FOR YOUR LIFE" . She is passionate about seeing believers know their worth and understand who they are in Christ. Cristina has discovered her calling and purpose in life and wants the same for others. She wants to help new believers grow in maturity in Christ. She currently works in a disability care home.

Other Books She Has Written

~God's Perfect Will For Your Life: God
Will Lead You To The Right Path

~Declare and Proclaim God's Word Over Your
Life: There Is Power In The Word Of God.

~Spreek En Verkondig Gods Woord Over Uw
Leven: Er Is Kracht In Het Woord Van God.

~Seven Things God Hates: Become The Person
That God Has Intended You To Be.

~Praying God's Word Over Your Children: God
Will Bring To Pass What He Has Spoken.

~Break Curses And Receive God's Blessings : Jesus Christ
Will Release You From The Chains On Your Hands.

~31 Days Of Spiritual And Personal Growth Devotional
: Becoming The Person God Created You To Be

~Pray God's Perfect Will For Your Life: Take
Your Prayer Life To The Next Level

~ Bid God's Volmaakte Wil Voor Je Leven:
Versterk Je Gebedsleven.

~ Zeven Dingen Die Voor God Een Gruwel Zijn:
Keer Af Van De Dingen Die God Veracht

~Siete Cosas Que Dios Detesta: Aléjese De
las Cosas Que Dios Desprecia.

~Sete Coisas Que Deus Detesta: Afastar-
se Das Coisas Que Deus Despreza.

For questions and testimonies go to:

Email: LivinginthewillofGod@hotmail.com

Facebook: https://www.facebook.com/CristinaDomingoss

ॐ

"At the end of the ten days, Daniel and his three friends looked healthier and better nourished than the young men who had been eating the food assigned by the king. So after that, the attendant fed them only vegetables instead of the food and wine provided for the others."

– Daniel 1:15–16 NLT